THE WAY OF BALANCE

The Way of Balance

A Natural Approach to Solar & Lunar Rhythms

Michelle Bouchard, L.Ac.

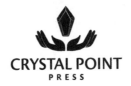

CRYSTAL POINT
PRESS

Tunnel Press, Ltd.
3589 Menoher Blvd.
Johnstown PA 15905

ISBN 978-0-941461-02-3 (paperback)
978-0-941461-13-9 (eBook)

Editor
    Kate Blake

Cover and text design
    Troy Scott Parker, Cimarron Design

Author photo
    Park O. Cover

Line art
    Steve Meraz

To my parents, Rose & Bert Bouchard

*My Dad taught me that everything is possible
and that humans are inherently good*

*My Mom was my first patient and
always believed in me and my medicine*

*And to the myriad of people who have
trusted me to help guide their health*

CONTENTS

INTRODUCTION   9

Spring   17

Summer   27

Late Summer   35

Fall   45

Winter   55

The New Moon   65

The Full Moon   73

ADDITIONAL RESOURCES   81

ABOUT THE AUTHOR   83

INTRODUCTION

My background as an acupuncturist and yoga teacher has afforded me a unique glimpse into the world of health and what it really takes to heal. But my true nature, the thing that drives me to help others is an overwhelming belief in the capability of our intuition, our *knowing* when things aren't quite right, our incredible strength, and the immense courage we possess to set things right. I am a naturalist at heart. When I have a headache or almost any other type of ache, I do not run to the medicine cabinet for ibuprofen. I question the existence of the headache, and I look for simple solutions as a remedy. *"Did I get enough rest?" "Do I need exercise?" "Is it something I ate?"* Those things are quantifiable. Fixable— in a natural sense. Our body gives us clues, each and every day, about how best to maintain and treat it. We really need to stop and listen.

> *To live in alignment, to follow and flow*
> *with the cycles of the natural order*
> *is an easier path for living.*

Going against nature's rhythms has long been part of modern man's need to control. In fact, our modern lifestyle is testament to our desire to control nature. The invention of electricity, being able to control personal climate (hot in winter, cold in summer), using up fossil fuels, our plentiful conveniences, are examples of upsetting the delicate balance that is our birthright. By studying the seasons, the rhythm of the Earth as it turns around the Sun, and the rhythm of the Moon as it turns around our planet, we can begin to take back our lives and once again find harmony.

The pandemic in 2020 has served to level the playing field. The experience has been stressful to so many. It has forced us to slow down and pay attention. Humans have begun to awaken and take advantage of new opportunities to pay attention to the planet and to what is natural.

Instead of flowing against the stream of life,
we have a chance to flow with it.

I am reminded of how timely these writings are as they offer a way to achieve this. I wrote this book with an underlying need to help you, the reader, know what you are up against. The knowledge I have gained in more than 20 years of being a Chinese medicine practitioner, an acupuncturist, and yoga teacher has allowed me a rare opportunity to learn from my personal challenges as well as from those of my patients and students. I have witnessed that the choices we make in how we live our lives can contribute to pain and suffering. Along the way, I have tried to teach myself and my students an easier way.

The natural world is our greatest teacher. She is our greatest ally, should we choose to stop and listen. This collection has served as a reminder to me of the long road I have also taken to live more harmoniously in society and in the natural world. Within the lunar and solar cycles, we also have our own life cycles. There is *Spring* in our lives, where everything is new and fresh. It is our *New Moon* time. Conversely, there is *Winter* when an old way of being dies or when we die. If we learn to recognize and honor the phase of life we are currently in, we get a chance to be more comfortable. We learn to flow with the seasons of our lives.

In order for you to fully grasp the Chinese medicine concepts I use here, I must first explain a bit of its background. The first concept you must understand is yin and yang.

It is the balance of all life. As seen through the eyes
of Chinese philosophy, yin and yang live in relation
to one another; neither of them is absolute. Loosely
translated, the yin aspect is the feminine component; the
darker, cold, inactive side. The yang aspect, is the male
component. It is the active, hot, bright side. The yin
can only appear to be cold in relation to something that
is yang, or hot. Lukewarm water, for instance, is yang
in comparison to cold water, which would be yin. But
lukewarm water is yin in comparison to hot water, which
would be considered yang. Lukewarm water also carries
within it the ability to change into its opposition. There
is a bit of cold in the water that would make it less hot.
Also, there is a bit of warm in the water that would make
it less cool. It can seem complex. Suffice it to say that yin
and yang are related to each other and rely on each other
to be defined. It is within the harmony of the aspects
of yin and yang and the laws of balance that Chinese
medicine gets its sacred wisdom.

*The idea is that the natural world is always
trying to seek a state of balance. Balance and
living in harmony are the ultimate goal.*

My intention as I write this is to help ignite curiosity
within you about where *you* live. I hope to spark a
questioning of and a fascination with the natural world
through *your* eyes. What is the area where you like to
live? Is it hot and dry? Cool and damp? Is it a combination
of these elements at different times and in different
seasons? In what ways can you honor the elements and
learn to live in balance?

Another definition is chi (also spelled qi). Chi is our
life force. Chi is the energy that drives us on a daily basis.
If our chi is low, we are not able to do very much, or as
much as if our chi is balanced. Chi is something that is
studied and quantifiable within the confines of Chinese
medicine. Chi is what we are trying to access and balance
through the mechanics of acupuncture when we place
thin needles along a particular meridian, or pathway,
in the body. Chi is by no means the only aspect we are
looking to balance. We are also attempting to balance
blood. In relation to blood, chi is yang; blood is yin.
Blood in Chinese medicine is similar to the bright red
liquid stuff that you know from scraping your arm. In
terms of Chinese medicine, it is also a vital component

to a healthy operating system. Chi and blood work synergistically and compartmentally to make you uniquely you.

I define a meridian as a pathway, or highway, along particular routes in your body. When there is pain or disease, a Chinese practitioner will say that a meridian is blocked, much like an accident on a highway. That practitioner will work to clean up the accident and clear the highway.

Through the practice of acupuncture and Chinese herbology, a Chinese medical practitioner is constantly and untiringly looking for ways to put you in balance. What distinguishes Chinese medicine from Western medicine is an underlying philosophy that a person's body is seeking balance. Whereas Western understanding operates from the principle that the system is already broken and seeks to remedy the broken aspect, Chinese medical understanding looks deeper at the entire system of brokenness. Why did it break? What structural aspect can we work on so it will not break again? Was the chi too weak? Was it too strong? What can we do to bring the system back to its natural state of balance? In what ways can we work with the natural rhythms that already exist for optimal health? A Chinese medical practitioner will take time to discuss many important lifestyle factors

that Western medicine may overlook—diet, activity
levels, sleep, digestion, environmental influences, and
stress levels, for example.

In this same spirit, this book was born. It is my humble
and extensive understanding of yet another component
of lifestyle. What is happening in the natural world?
Can and will we work with the natural rhythms in the
seasonal systems that surround and guide us? Should we
stop and listen? Because I live in Western Pennsylvania,
I often hear my patients says things like, *"Boy, I hate this
rain." "Winter is the worst season." "Summer is my favorite
time of the year."* Since adopting a more natural approach
to the seasons, as they come, when they come, I have
found within myself the ease and comfort of a life that
is lived honestly and more balanced. It is my sincere
hope that you learn and adopt a better understanding of
nature's cycles and how they impact our bodies so that
you may live more harmoniously.

A quick word about my point of reference. I live
in the northern hemisphere of the globe. I live in the
United States—specifically in the northeast. The same
principles that apply to me may be the exact opposite for
you, seasonally. My summer months of June, July, and
August might be your winter months. My cold, snowy
winter may be mild if you live in the southern United

States. This book is only a *guide*—an exploration, if you will, into your particular understanding of the seasons and climate in your area. The moon aspects remain consistent but understand that people across the globe are experiencing them at different times.

As a healer, I specialize in helping you heal yourself—when you are ready. It is my intention to help you get to your next level of health. I love this job. I get to witness miracles. I have studied the deep layers of healing involved in creating miracles for others. There are many layers of dis-ease. This book is a dive into one more layer—environmental. The place where we live, the seasons, and the world around us shape our experience of true health. We have an opportunity to honor the changing world around us by learning to live and flow with it. Chinese medicine, as I have learned, is a system of balance. Cold herbs treat fevers. Hot food warms us during cold months. There is a continual dance we play in our ever-evolving world. The one truth is this: There is continual change. Day turns to night. Winter turns to Spring. We have the chance to allow these changes to guide us gently as we learn to walk this balance.

– Michelle Bouchard, L.Ac.
Ligonier, Pennsylvania

Spring

The budding of the trees is one of the first signs of Spring on the horizon. The Spring equinox, i.e., Vernal equinox, represents that exact moment when the time of light and the time of dark are equal. Trees and plants carry within their cells unique understanding that around this time, it is safe again to open their budding flowers and leaves to the world. After the Spring equinox, the lightness will prevail. Warmth will inevitably follow.

Another sign of the arrival of Spring is increased activity of the natural world. Birds come back from their winter homes or places of hibernation. They begin to sing their mating songs and gather up materials for building summer homes. Bears and larger animals come out of hiding, and Mother Nature provides the climate and circumstances for mating so that baby animals are born. Everything in nature takes on a brighter, greener, shinier hue. As I walk along the streets of my town in

Pennsylvania, I see the buds on the trees bursting forth. I see squirrels and chipmunks scurry about with an urgency of preparation and welcoming. Flowers begin to boldly sprout from their winter hiding. Some of them, having gotten too excited by one warmer day may open too soon, before the last frost, and lose their lives to an untimely demise. Yet, somehow there is a perfect balance unfolding in Spring, and you can almost hear Mother Nature breathe as plants pop up from the ground.

People too, have a natural enthusiasm and excitement around this time that speaks to their own awakenings. As a reflection of nature, they too will sometimes leave their house with great enthusiasm for warmth, only to be greeted to continued cold, albeit not as cold! It always amuses me to see people in the North wearing shorts in March! Sleep patterns in people begin to change, ever so slightly, as the need for sleep becomes less. With more amounts of daylight, the natural rhythm becomes less involved in hunkering down, staying warm, and being inactive.

In the Spring, I often find myself waking bright and early, not quite with, but almost with the Sun. I find myself being able to take longer, more frequent walks, and of course, I begin to spend time in the garden. After what feels like never-ending Winter, I begin to explore more gardens and wooded areas. Without the blanket of snow on the ground, I get a chance to really feel the ground, the earth, beneath my feet. If the temperatures are warm enough, putting my bare feet in the soil brings me peace and healing. The awakening of the natural world mirrors in me a belief that *I get a chance to start anew.*

As plants begin to sprout, our natural inclination is to want to start eating lighter, greener. Spring greens: spinach, lettuce, asparagus, and arugula take center stage. Unlike the heaviness of Winter, most Spring greens can be eaten raw, as our digestion begins to awake and refresh. This is a normal cleansing process that helps us restart. The taste of Spring, according to Chinese medicine, is sour. One of Mother Nature's treats at this time are dandelions, which are quite bitter and extraordinarily cleansing, especially for the liver. Spring is the season of detoxification. According to our man-made calendar, January 1st is the day many people set as the beginning of dieting and trying to lose weight. However, according to nature's rhythms, Spring is the better time to accomplish this goal. Our diets become easier and leaner, and our activity levels begin to increase.

The yin organ that we focus on strengthening in Chinese medicine is the liver. Its corresponding yang organ is the gall bladder. The liver is responsible for the smooth flow of chi, our innate energy. To accomplish the task of helping our chi to flow smoothly, the liver is responsible for the expression of our emotions, particularly anger. The gall bladder, according to Chinese medicine, is responsible for decision making. When anger and frustration get pent up and stuck inside of us, Chinese medicine says that the liver has become stagnant. Regular exercise, a cleaner diet, and the full expression of all of our emotions can really support the function of our liver and gall bladder in keeping energy freely moving.

In our American culture, the true expression of the range of emotions is not easily accomplished. Women, in particular, are taught to almost never express anger; while men are taught that anger is almost the only acceptable emotion. In fact, many men are not encouraged to explore the wide range of emotions, and they end up defaulting to the only one they know— anger. Women are taught to hold in anger, almost to the point of it becoming its own driving force that gets expressed inappropriately. Women are not taught how to stand up for themselves in a fight. As a result, women's anger often gets turned inward and can lead to depression, low self-esteem, anxiety, and in severe cases, mania. Lessons that little girls learn early involve quieting their inner frustrations for the sake of the greater good. Little boys are often taught and encouraged to get physical with their anger. When other emotions come up, like grief or sadness, boys are taught to "man up" and hold it in.

From my experience as a Chinese medicine practitioner, liver chi stagnation is probably the most common condition I address. I realize my interpretation of the issue around anger expression can appear primitive and quite general, but time and time again I see the same themes arise in my patients and in my own family systems. The pressures of our modern, hectic, fast-paced world create stress. Simply put,

Stress translates to liver chi stagnation.

Manifestations of liver chi stagnation seen in a clinical setting include, but are not limited to depression, anxiety, uncontrollable anger, menstrual irregularities, and muscle fatigue or tightness. Stress, in a general sense, is the number one predictor of chronic illness. Autoimmune diseases, where the body's own defense mechanisms go haywire, are a direct by-product of the stressful lives we have created or allow to be created for ourselves. Any other forms of stress reduction on a broad level are powerful to help avoid disease. Think along the lines of slowing down, maybe meditation, yoga, chi gong, or tai chi. Literally, the word *tai* is translated as *big*. Chi is what I have been talking about in terms of life force, or internal energy flow. When a person practices tai chi, the idea is to cultivate and build big energy. I have not met anyone yet who does not want more energy. Think about it.

So how can we support the liver? First and foremost, we can allow for the true and pure expression of all our emotions. Physical movement, in particular, helps the chi to move within the body. Chi and blood move together, and when the heart is pumping blood more adequately and swiftly, the chi will also begin to move. Did you ever notice that when you are feeling extremely low energy, a brisk 15- or 20-minute walk will bring up your energy level? It almost seems counterintuitive—that expending energy by walking produces more energy. Extended, regular, exercise is probably one of the best treatments for depression.

Along with movement, there are a wide range of Chinese herbs that are helpful to move liver chi. I was not kidding about eating dandelions. Dandelion root is called Pu Gong Yin; it is an excellent herb to help move a stagnant or stuck liver meridian. However, the easiest

most common sources are the domestic foods we eat.
Start noticing more sour foods and foods that begin to
sprout in your garden or yard. Arugula comes to mind
along with kale, celery, asparagus, dandelion flowers,
spinach, and collard greens. Put a few drops of lemon
in your water first thing in the morning. All of these
foods will naturally help you clean out and freshen up
the liver. Even in our American culture, we understand
that it is important to detoxify the liver. Heavy alcohol
consumption, along with heavy sugar and fat intake, will
wreak havoc on the liver.

Also, something that is not talked about enough is
the overuse of medications. Everything that is foreign
to the body, meaning anything that cannot be found in
nature, needs to get processed through the blood in the
liver. The heavy use of pesticides in our food sources as
well, ends up getting dumped into the liver. If you are
using pesticides or herbicides in your garden, I invite you
to explore natural and life-sustaining alternatives. Our
bodies were not designed to assimilate the plethora of
harsh chemicals that are currently found in our water
and food supplies. Anything you can do to help move
along the chi of your liver meridian is helpful.

Another function of the liver is to store blood;
therefore, we see menstrual problems with chi

stagnation. A different function involves relaxing and controlling sinews. The sinews include joints and tendons, and it is the job of the liver meridian to regulate either contraction or relaxation, primarily in relation to the blood. Therefore, on a clinical level, we see muscle fatigue, weakness, tightness, or lack of control. Think of leg cramps or restless leg syndrome, for instance. Because every organ system works in direct relation with other organ systems, we also will see digestive disturbances which are controlled by the spleen and stomach meridians. Manifestations include, but are not limited to, belching, acid reflux, vomiting or nausea, and diarrhea. These manifestations can sometimes exist completely on their own when spleen and stomach chi is weak or deficient. However, the added impact of the unsupported liver/gall bladder is quite harmful.

What practical steps can we take during Spring and this time of new energy?

* Begin to add Spring greens to your diet, Yes, it is time to wake up the digestive system again after a long, cold, sluggish winter of heavy eating.

* Start more movement. 15–20 minutes of sustained movement is excellent to clear stagnation in the

meridian. Before you tell me that you worked for 20 minutes in the garden, I will remind you that your blood needs to be pumping regularly, not sporadically. Garden work does not qualify.

* Along those lines, get out in nature! Mother Nature is inviting you to join her in her awakening.

* Less sleep is o.k. I almost never say this, so take advantage when I do! Your normal sleep rhythms might appear to shorten when Spring arrives.

* If you have fallen off the wagon with your New Year's resolutions, Spring is an excellent time to refresh and restart.

* Along those lines, Spring is the best time to revisit your diet, particularly if you are trying to lose weight.

* Some lemon in water, first thing in the morning, is ideal for cleaning the liver and waking up your digestive system.

* Spring is an excellent time to plant seeds. I see this both in a literal sense and in a metaphorical sense. What in your life are you wanting to grow?

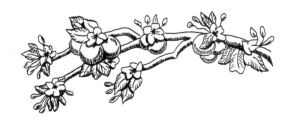

Summer

Who doesn't love Summer? In the Northern
Hemisphere, after Winter has dragged us down with its
cold and darkness, Summer comes along and is a breath
of fresh air. In relation to Winter, the polar opposite of
Summer, we have a chance to be active and extroverted.
If Winter is the ultimate yin, or inward time, Summer is
the ultimate yang, or active time. We sleep less; we move
more; we soak in the goodness of the sun with its eternal
brightness and warmth. As I write this I am sitting out on
my front porch, open to the new day and all that it will
bring. With children getting a break from school, families
go on vacations, where there is much laughter and fun.
(Okay, ideally there is much laughter and fun. I've been
on a few family getaways that were not so much fun.)
Swimming, boating, gardening, and just spending time
with others are some of the many activities you will see
people enjoying in the Summer.

Summer is the pure expression of joy and happiness, according to Chinese medicine. When was the last time you felt joyful? Is there a memory that includes a summertime activity? A bigger question, and one that is not often asked in Western culture, is *"What brings you joy?"* Your answer does not have to include an outward activity. Sitting on the front porch and reading a good book may bring you joy. Curling up with a favorite pet may bring you joy. In our hectic, fast-paced culture one of the first questions people ask one another is, *"What do you do?"* But if you stop and notice, when children meet each other they ask more important questions, like *"What is your favorite color?"* or, *"What is your favorite TV show?"* These questions dig deeper into the heart of an underlying exploration of our inner joy—what lights us up. If you have not explored these answers in a while, summertime may be your time!

The corresponding meridian associated with Summer and our expression of joy is the heart meridian. Our heart meridian is responsible for pumping blood, just like in Western medicine, but it also has the unique role of housing the actions and activities of the mind. Some ancients believed the heart meridian was the most important of all, calling it the ruler of all the internal organs. Think about it; if the heart is not strong and healthy, blood does not get moved to the organs. A person with weak heart chi lacks blood and strength and will appear fragile and pale. At the same time, if the heart chi is deficient, a person's mental capacity is compromised. This is when you see mental disorders come into play. Schizophrenia, mania, psychosis, depression, anxiety, and a host of other mental imbalances are manifestations of problems with the heart meridian. Seen this way, a strong, healthy heart is perhaps the single most important meridian. Strong body. Strong mind.

The related yang meridian associated with the heart is the small intestine. As in Western anatomy, the small intestine is responsible for separating the food and drink that we ingest into nutrition to fuel our bodies and waste to be discarded. In this respect, the heart and small intestine work synergistically to separate and clarify our mind. Decision making, as in making good decisions versus making poor decisions, is largely a function of the small intestine meridian. This is not to be confused with decision making that is fueled by the meridian of the gall bladder (the yang aspect of the yin organ, liver.) While the gall bladder gives us the courage and wherewithal to actually *make* a decision, the small intestine clears our mind and makes way for the *discernment of making the best decision.* In this respect the yin/yang organ pair of the heart and small intestine work on a much deeper level of a healthy mind.

When Chinese medicine talks about functions of the mind, it is referring to a concept called *shen*. Shen has many meanings, but one that resonates profoundly with me includes this quote:

> **Shen is the light that shines out of a person's eyes when they are truly awake.**

Conversely, when the shen is imbalanced or disturbed, a person's mental capacity is just *off* somehow. Shen encompasses the entire range of our emotional, mental, and spiritual aspects of thought. It is what makes us uniquely human. The heart is responsible for balanced and healthy shen. Along with our conscious thought, the heart governs our unconscious thought also. Therefore, good sleep is a function and a barometer of balanced shen. Too much sleep or not enough can both cause and be a function of imbalanced shen. Dreaming, also, is controlled by aspects of a healthy heart. Excessive dreaming or nightmares indicate heart imbalance. When the heart meridian is healthy, the mind does not float around at night and a person will be able to get to sleep and stay asleep easily, with a normal amount of dreaming.

The condition of the heart also affects and controls speech. Abnormalities may result in stuttering or aphasia, which literally means, *without speech*. Talking and laughing are included in this function. If a person's shen is out of balance, you will notice excessive talking or excessive non-talking if the person is depressed, or uncontrollable or inappropriate laughter, (think mania). For me, this is particularly interesting in light of the fact that the emotion of the heart meridian which is most manifest in the Summer, is that of joy. Excessive joy or uncontrollable laughter can sometimes be pathological from a Chinese medical perspective. Also, expressions of joy may not always be outward. Joy may come from floating in a pool, which is considered inactive, or inward.

What is also interesting to me is the function of sleep from a Chinese medical perspective. Winter is naturally a time of the most amount of sleep, and yet Summer is a time of the least amount of sleep. So then, what constitutes a normal amount of sleep? I think it varies from person to person. But the questions you should be asking yourself, in relation to sleep time are: *"Am I waking up feeling rested?" "Do I have enough energy throughout my day?" "Do I need stimulants (caffeine, nicotine) to keep me going?"*

Sleep is probably one of our most underrated bodily functions. We absolutely need it to stay alive. Yet, as a culture, we often take getting good sleep for granted. Think of college days when you pulled *all-nighters* to crank out an important assignment. Think of the endless cups of coffee you drink just to feel human in the morning. For that matter, think of your afternoon coffee fixes, just so you could survive the second part of the day. Even our language around the topic of sleep is interesting. *"Yea, I can survive on only 4 or 5 hours of sleep a night"* is something I have heard more than once said in a boastful way. It fascinates me how little credence we give to the concept of the healthy need for good sleep. Surviving lack of sleep should not be considered a goal nor an accomplishment. We should be honoring our bodies' unique abilities to restore and reset themselves with proper amounts of sleep. We should be focused on a thriving and healthy system instead of a system we neglect and push to its limits. Having said that, yes, it is *normal* to sleep less in summertime. The Summer is absolute yang time, and sleep is a yin activity.

So with the lesser amount of sleep you are getting, think about what type of activities you enjoy during the Summer. Think about how best to fuel your body for those activities. The taste of Summer according to Chinese medicine is bitter. Kale, spinach, lettuces, cucumber, sprouts, wild mushrooms, lemons, and limes should all be a part of a healthy summer diet. This is the season for salads! With the outside temperatures blazing, it is o.k. and appropriate to add energetically cold, *i.e.*, raw, foods to your system. Watermelon is an excellent summertime treat. Fruits of all kinds should be part of a healthy summertime diet. Heavier foods, such as meats, cheeses, nuts, and grains should be kept to a minimum.

At the height of the most active time of year, as you think of the best ways to enjoy your Summer, here are a few tips and tricks I like to use to get the most out of this season.

* Do one thing each day that brings you joy. Although I would like to extend this opportunity and tell you to do this this all year long, summertime, in particular, is a good time to do things you enjoy.

* Eat healthy, clean, and light. More raw vegetables and fruits are appropriate and necessary to fuel you during this season.

* Continue to spend time in nature. Even if the days are hot, the mornings and evenings in Summer are a

wonderful time to enjoy the great outdoors. Tend to
your garden or just enjoy a walk.

* Be social. Summer is the ultimate expression of
yang, and as such, lends itself to gatherings with
others, big or small.

* Drink plenty of water. I cannot stress this enough.
Especially if the opportunity affords you the chance
to sweat during the heat of the day. And remember,
sweating is a natural and healthy process.

* Get good sleep. Particularly during Summer, when
the heart meridian is at its most vulnerable, sleep
helps us reset our minds. If your sleep is poor, your
mental activities will suffer. Concentration, focus,
attention to detail are all functions of a healthy
mind.

* Avoid heavy foods. Meats, dairy products, nuts,
legumes, and grains are all considered heavy and can
literally weigh you down during the Summer.

* Outward activities are more appropriate during
Summer. Biking, hiking, swimming, visiting with
friends, group activities, and group sports are
beneficial and healthy during the Summer.

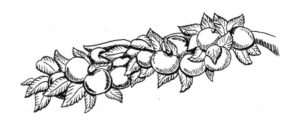

Late Summer

There really is not an equivalent of Late Summer
in Western understanding. Perhaps Indian Summer
comes the closest. It is when the days are still hot, like
in Summer, but the nights start to cool down, and even
a frost or two happens. It is the utmost season of vast
harvest, as the fall and winter vegetables start coming
out—squashes, pumpkins, gourds. The days still can
remain hot though, sometimes insufferable. Where I live,
people continue to run their air conditioners throughout
the day, and perhaps because they forgot to turn them
off, through the night. Animals feel the shift in earth
energy and begin to migrate to warmer destinations.
How do they know it is time? My guess is that they pay
attention to the signs. As I witness Late Summer where
I am, I am saddened by the abrupt disappearance of the
hummingbirds at the feeder. Yet, wherever their desti-
nation, I am sure they are also being welcomed home.

In Chinese medicine theory, Late Summer honors and supports the energy of the spleen and stomach meridians. The spleen meridian is the yin aspect of the two; the stomach is the yang. Both meridians are responsible for the breakdown of the foods we eat into nourishment to sustain life. To a lesser degree, the two meridians also help regulate fluid metabolism. The spleen is also responsible for holding blood in place. If there is an imbalance of the spleen meridian, a woman may have excessive menstrual blood. The amount of usable energy and stamina to carry out tasks on any given day is directly related to the healthy function of the spleen and stomach. So too does our muscle tone directly correlate. The way that I think of them is as akin to an image of *holding things in place* and nourishing our systems by transforming our food to usable energy.

On that note, I would like to take a moment to discuss the importance of a healthy diet. The food we take into our bodies is literally fuel for our systems to work. If you want your body to perform better, feed it better fuel. While I am human and succumb to the occasional not-so-healthy treat, I do it with the understanding that I may pay a later price for said indulgence. I do it only sparingly.

Over 10 years ago I figured out for myself that my body is allergic to wheat. Specifically, the gluten in wheat. While I would like nothing better than to wake up in the morning and pop some bread into the toaster for breakfast, I do not do that. I recognize and honor the limitations of my own system. How did I figure out my allergy? Well—I got sick. Digestive system sick. The food I was putting into my stomach was coming back out at night as diarrhea.

My body was trying to tell me something. I visited a gastroenterologist (in Western medicine this is a stomach doctor) who told me I had irritable bowel syndrome, IBS. I was sent home with a prescription for medicine *to slow down my intestines.* I left his office with more questions than answers. How did he know it was IBS when the visit lasted less than 5 minutes? How long would I need to take this particular medicine? Were there any tests to rule out another diagnosis?

The short version of the story is that I did not take the medicine. It did not make sense to me. It did not *feel* right in my gut. I am not trying to make any puns here. I prayed and asked for a different answer. One morning, after sitting in my meditation, I got my answer. Laying on the floor next to my meditation pillow was a book about Chinese medicine and eating healthy. (For your reference this is included for additional reading at the end of this book.) I opened the book randomly, and it opened up to the page on celiac disease. I had every symptom listed as a disfunction of celiac disease—or a gluten sensitivity. This *felt* right. It felt (in my gut) that this was the warning and solution my body was giving me. I stopped eating wheat. After only one day, my symptoms started to go away. I tell you this story for two reasons. First, it is important to listen to your body and what your gut is telling you. Doctors do not have all the answers. One of the first questions I ask my patients is, *"What do you think is wrong?"*

You are the master and caretaker of your body.

Second, my symptoms were directly related to an unhealthy spleen/stomach meridian according to Chinese medicine principles. Had I ignored the messages my body was giving, or had I followed the advice of the gastroenterologist, I could have gotten much sicker than I already was. Digestion, and healthy digestion, is crucial to a healthy overall system.

So how does the spleen/stomach become damaged? The pathogenic influence to avoid in order to maintain a healthy spleen is dampness. This dampness can be either external, as in living in a damp environment, or internal, as in eating too many sugary, mucous-forming foods.

Because the spleen is responsible for transforming the food we eat, diet plays an important role in helping to regulate energy. Damp becomes problematic when the foods we eat are also too cold. By this I mean energetically cold. Raw foods, over time, can harm the spleen. Drinks with ice are considered very damaging to the spleen. When dampness is able to penetrate and weaken the spleen, a person will suffer from prolonged periods of fatigue. The transformation that occurs in the intestines will suffer as well, and a person will feel bloated and most likely suffer from loose stools. Beyond the types of food we eat, Chinese medicine also points out the importance of eating in moderation (stopping before you are full), eating without distractions (no eating on the go), and staying away from fad diets.

The taste of the spleen/stomach meridian is sweet. With a very large note of caution: I urge you to explore what true sweetness entails. A tomato is sweet, naturally. Candy, on the other hand, is made from refined cane sugar which most likely does not grow in your back yard and is processed to make it the white powdery stuff you know. Fruit is naturally sweet. Soda is sweetened with sugar, or goddess forbid, unnatural sweetener. Always choose cane sugar over chemical-based sweeteners such as aspartame. I am not going too far down this path, but if you are still using artificial sugar-like products, or *diet* drinks sweetened with them, I encourage you to research the medical problems associated with them—diabetes and kidney disease for instance.

The *sweet* in relation to helping the spleen/stomach meridian is a *natural* sweet. Carrots are naturally sweet. If you do not immediately think of a carrot as being sweet, I challenge you to try a glass of carrot juice. Are sweets (as in candy and soda) something you crave? Take a moment and ask yourself, *"What is sweet in my life?"* Maybe your dog brings you sweetness. Maybe it is your children.

I have already mentioned some foods which are beneficial during Late Summer. Diving into a bigger list, I would include millet, corn, cabbage, garbanzo beans, squash, potatoes, string beans, soybeans, sweet potatoes, rice, peas, and chestnuts. Avoid mucous-forming foods. Dairy products, except small amounts of butter, excessive raw foods, unnaturally sweet foods, oily foods, and heavy meals all encourage mucous formation. It is also important to stay away from highly processed or chemically treated foods. Avoid late night eating and overeating in general. Also make sure that your meals do not contain too many ingredients in one sitting. Anything you can do to ease the burden of digestion is helpful.

The emotional component connected to the spleen is over-thinking—sometimes bordering on obsessiveness. I always equate it to deep worry. By over-thinking or analyzing a situation too intensely, we can cause great harm to the spleen. Students in college sometimes suffer spleen damage from having to balance their lives between work and play. People who sit at a desk all day are not only harming their cardiovascular health, but also their digestive health. Our bodies were made to move around, and a sedentary life is not good on many levels.

I am definitely a person who worries. What is fascinating to me about over thinking and worrying is that it solves nothing. There is literally nothing that gets accomplished from worrying over things. When I meet a patient who over-thinks, I start inquiring about digestion. It is always interesting to me what some people consider *normal* in terms of healthy digestion. Bowel elimination, at least once a day, with well formed stools is considered healthy. Anything other than that is grounds for examining the energy of the spleen/stomach meridian, and to a lesser extent the large intestine meridian.

I touched on the topic of constipation earlier, but it is worth examining further so you can see how it is understood energetically. Yes, there are some basic and easy measures you can take to overcome constipation. These are things you should be doing anyway such as drinking water, eating a variety of fruits and vegetables, exercising, and stretching; are all excellent ways to naturally combat constipation.

Worry or over-thinking or obsessiveness is also important when looking at the physical phenomenon of constipation. There are also psychological components of constipation. Not being *able to let go* of things. Holding on to grudges, the past, or hoarding things. When obsessive thinking becomes out of control it can lead to constipation. Your body's natural inclination is to get rid of waste products, but when your mind is holding on to things, the spillover may take root in your bodily functions. In every case of constipation, the solution is not always the same, but learning how *to let go* will serve you well. (Letting go is addressed in the Full Moon chapter.)

During this bonus season of Late Summer with the weather staying hot throughout the day, the following ideas can help you ensure a healthy spleen/stomach meridian and healthy digestion.

* Limit your intake of ice in drinks. I am not telling you to do away with cold drinks altogether. I am recommending that ice in drinks is considered too cold. Limit them.

* Enjoy the beginning of late harvests. Certain vegetables and fruits are at their peak during this late summer season. Broccoli, kale, and brussels sprouts do well when the nights are cold, and days are hot.

* Check your over-thinking. Are you prone to worry? Does worrying help you? Worry leads to anxiety and other psychological issues. As much as you can, limit the amount of worrying you do.

* Pay attention to and honor your digestion. Is there something you can do right now to honor how your digestion works? Is there something you should avoid that you are not?

* If you are a person who has not yet developed letting go skills, maybe you could learn some simple yoga postures that could help. (Refer to the Full Moon chapter).

* If you are a student or studying something intense, make sure that you are taking regular breaks throughout your study time.

* Continue to enjoy the wonders of nature. You may have noticed this as a theme throughout the book. When you really pay attention to the natural world, you are already living in better balance and better harmony.

* Bring yourself sweetness. Without overdoing it on sugary snacks, maybe try a smoothie? Maybe buy yourself some flowers? Maybe play yourself a sweet song?

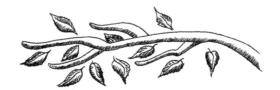

Fall

Fall. Autumn. The time of harvest and the beginning
of the descent to the most yin time—Winter. The very
word, *fall*, implies a "letting go energy" as we watch the
leaves on the trees change and drop to their death. They
are a superior reminder to us of the impermanence
of life. Gardens have been or are being harvested,
and abundance is the energy. People are busy storing
(freezing in our modern culture) and canning their
harvests. Fall is the time when the Native Americans
and Pilgrims came together in America to rejoice and to
celebrate their bountiful crops. It was also the time, and
should still be the time, when we are looking ahead to
meeker bounty, when we must rely on the foods we store
to sustain us through the days of Winter.

So much of the experience of the everyday American
has become disconnected from this local earth rhythm
of harvest because many people live in cities and suburbs

where we have access to an *international market* that
provides us fresh produce, fruits, and staples from other
countries. While I am grateful to have such abundant
access to food from all over the world, I wonder what
kind of impact we are making on sustainability. Notice
what is local in your own grocery stores. Notice what
has travelled far to end up on your plate. At what cost
do we acquire food internationally? I hope by now you
are gaining a better awareness that the foods we eat each
season are usually grown *in* that season. Just because
we have international access to watermelon in Winter
does not mean it is good for us if we eat it in Winter.
Over time, large populations of people have adapted and
adjusted what they eat to what was available. I think of
my ancestors who came from Canada where the Winters
are cold and harsh. Some of the recipes that have been
handed down from them reflect an increased emphasis
on animal fats. They used what was available, and it
served them in maintaining warmth.

As I look around there is one animal I see over and
over again. He/she is a reminder to me of how we must
plan ahead for what is coming next. The squirrel scurries
and gathers and stores acorns and nuts. I have noticed
in the past that when the squirrels leave acorns lying
around, the Winter turns out to be rather mild. With an

inner sense of knowing what's ahead, the animals who are preparing for the next season show and guide me, if I pay attention. This Fall I have not noticed an abundance of acorns, and the squirrel activity has been quite frantic, attempting to store away what is available and abundant. I am also thinking ahead, of indoor projects and more inward activities, like reading and writing, that I can start during this season. I hear people get disgruntled when the weather turns colder. They instinctively know what is ahead and are dreading it. The days are beginning to shorten as well, and Summer activities are arrested due to the cold and dark energies moving in. I encourage you to enjoy this "gathering nuts" energy. Plan ahead and begin to rejoice in the balanced energy of slowing down.

Fall is the yang going into the yin, in Chinese medicine. It is the season of dryness and the lung meridian. The lung takes chi from the air and mixes it with the chi, or life force, obtained from food. The lung has an immune enhancing function of keeping our systems moistened to ward off invasion from viruses. This is particularly interesting to me this year as our world is in the middle of a global pandemic and the coronavirus has killed so many. This Fall there is expected to be another wave of outbreaks resulting in more loss of human life. But this pattern of illness, flu, and viral outbreaks happens every year during the Fall.

So, what can we do to support the lung meridian? How can we live in harmony during this season for optimal immunity? Lung health, according to Chinese medicine, is directly correlated to our ability to easily *let go*. Grief is the emotion connected with the lung meridian, and it is the strength of the lung meridian that allows us to process the physical, emotional, and spiritual *letting go* of things, people, and situations. The corresponding yang organ that works together with the lung is the large intestine. Like it does in Western understanding, the large intestine clears out waste and that which is no longer needed. People with a strong lung/large intestine constitution have the ability *to hold on to* their principles and keep their commitments. At the same time, they *let go* of relationships or situations that no longer serve them without carrying resentment or repressing the associated grief needed in order to do so. The act of focusing internally (living in harmony with this season) helps to clear and disperse lung chi, and the lung then has the ability to drive out potential disease. Healthy bowel function, too, is directly correlated. People who tend to *hold on* too tightly, or do not allow the process of *letting go* end up with poor elimination function and disease. The simple act of breathing, with an intentional purpose of processing stored emotion, particularly grief, does wonders in restoring and promoting healthy lung/large intestine chi.

The taste associated with Fall is pungent. That is a difficult taste to understand with our Western minds. In general, I think of foods that are moistening and slightly sour. Think fermented foods such as sauerkraut, pickles, sourdough bread, cheese, and yogurt. A small amount of these foods goes a long way. This time of year means that it is time to start cooking your foods again. The summer salad days are over. The days of Fall are dry normally, and to balance the outward dryness, add some moistening foods, particularly fruit, to your diet. Apples, pears, persimmon, loquat come into season and are excellent lung tonics. Other moistening foods include soybean products, millet, barley, pinenuts, peanuts, honey, rice syrup, eggs, clams, crab, oysters, mussels, herring, and pork. Of course, this list is just a sampling of the many wonderful foods for Fall.

Just a short note about dairy products. Fall is a good time for dairy products, provided you are not allergic, and your system is strong enough. Milk from a cow was made for baby cows. Baby cows have four stomachs. Humans do not. It is amazing to me that an entire industry grew up around milking these large gentle animals. If you do not know whether or not you are allergic to dairy products, try going without them for a month or two and see how you feel.

Dryness is something to pay attention to in the Fall. By dryness, I mean that the person's skin is consistently dry—dry hair, cracked and brittle nails, dry throat, usually thin body, dry cough, and itchiness. In fact, itchy skin is another condition of dry and deficient lung chi. Skin overall is ruled by the lung and large intestine meridian. Any type of deficiency can result in a myriad of lung conditions—psoriasis, hives, eczema. While Western medicine does not always have good answers for skin problems, Chinese medicine can look at the other components of weak lung/large intestine chi. Is this person eating enough moistening foods? Do they have a dry constitution? Is there underlying grief? Is this person eliminating toxins well? Is this person's environment too dry? When I lived on the western slope of Colorado, which is essentially a desert, I witnessed more lung deficiency and the resulting problems of a dry external environment. My patients would sometimes show up with a dry, unproductive cough. Dry nails, skin, and hair was also common. Shortness of breath is another symptom of weak lung chi.

One more note about healthy lung and large intestine function follows. A sedentary lifestyle is incompatible with healthy respiration and elimination. Our systems were not designed to go without breath. Our systems can go days or weeks without water. We can go weeks or months without food. We cannot go more than a few minutes without breath. Honor your breath and your lungs for taking in the vital element of air. Do this by moving your body and allowing yourself to breathe hard and deep. In that same vein, the large intestines will work better when vital blood is brought to them through exercise. Obviously, the type of food you eat will also encourage and promote healthy bowel function.

Because I was born in the Fall, this time of year holds special magic for me. The leaves here in Western Pennsylvania are breathtaking as they change colors and drop. As a child, one of my dearest memories was raking leaves and jumping into the pile! Even as an adult, the smell of the fallen leaves and the sound of their crunch as I walk through my neighborhood brings a smile on my face. Something about the sunny Fall days and cool Fall nights brings me gentle comfort. I hope this gives you something to think about.

*Here is a brief list of how you can best
honor this wonderful Fall season.*

* Harvest all of the year's bounty. Pick vegetables and flowers from a garden. Canning and freezing at this time will help you participate and feel this great abundance.

* Keep exercising. Just because the weather may have turned cooler where you live, does not mean you stop moving. Bundle yourself up and get out there.

* Watch what the animals are doing in your area. I mentioned the squirrels racing around and storing nuts and seeds where I live. Turns out we are having a cold winter after all. They knew and were planning accordingly.

* Share the bounty of the season. If your harvest was abundant, share it with others. That was the original premise of Thanksgiving—honoring and sharing a large bounty. In our modern culture, it may look like donating to a particular charity or cause.

* Begin sleeping more. This is the season for hunkering down and cozying up.

* Switch to warm beverages. It is the time for hot tea and cocoa. To balance the coolness, drink and eat warm.

* Start slowing down. Fall is the season before Winter. We are beginning to move to stillness. Inside activities like reading, writing, and drawing are appropriate.

* Warming soups should be on the menu. As a direct balance of the cool in the air, start making soups and stews. Warming spices (think pumpkin spice) should be used at this time of year.

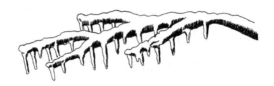

Winter

The dark, cold, season of Winter contains within it the energy of going inward. It is a season related to hibernation and going inside energetically. It is an ending. A death. However, as we know from this type of study by now, the end is just a pathway to a new beginning. One could not open to something new unless space is made for that new thing by letting go of something old. This is Winter—in all of her dark and cold finery.

In Chinese medicine, Winter is ruled by the energy of the kidney and urinary bladder meridian. Kidneys are the source of all life. Therefore, it is fitting that they embody the season associated with the end of life as well. The kidney meridian is responsible for normal reproductive function in Chinese medicine. The kidneys give rise, literally, to every other organ system and help us adapt to life at the base level, the root level. In fact, if you think of a tree as a metaphor for seasonal changes, the kidney and urinary bladder meridian would be the roots of the tree. Without them there would be no support. The kidneys are the yin aspect of the corresponding urinary bladder meridian, which is the yang aspect.

The sense of hearing is associated with the kidney meridian. The element of the kidneys is water. The emotion of the kidneys is fear. It is not entirely coincidental that we say things like, *"I was so scared I peed my pants."* In a very real sense, we can understand the fundamentals that make up these Winter organs.

What is the energy we need to cultivate in order to flow better with the season of Winter? If we look around us, we notice animals who are far less active. We see certain mammals hibernating for long periods during Winter. Most notably, bears hibernate. Other creatures, including our house pets, spend more time sleeping, less time eating, and less time moving about. Daylight hours are shorter, and our human demands for sleep increase naturally during Winter. Depending on your normal sleep pattern, the Winter holds a collective energy of heaviness and fatigue. Because the temperatures are colder, bundling up by a fire, drinking more hot drinks, and feeling less desire for outward activity is entirely appropriate.

Because mid-Winter marks the end of the calendar year in the Northern Hemisphere, reflection on the year is healthy. Activities such as reading or writing, maybe drawing, are appropriate during the Winter because these involve less physical energy and require us to keep our thoughts focused on our own experiences. Winter is an introvert's playground. Although people do engage in outdoor sports in Winter, the lack of sufficient Sun available in a day gives rise to more indoor activities. During Winter, I love to practice yoga and enjoy reading even more than the rest of the year. Winter months are good for yoga that is slow and healing. Restorative yoga, or yin yoga, are good choices. Tai chi is another great activity to cultivate in Winter.

I sit here wrapped in many layers of shirts and sweaters sipping hot tea. I am reminded of my shaman friend, who reminded me to wear socks in the Winter months. I have seen people go without socks when the temperature gets colder. This goes against all that is natural. We are not fur-based mammals! We need to be wearing heavier clothing and eating foods that are better aligned with nourishment and warmth. In fact, I might be one of the first people to tell you *not* to eat salads during Winter. In Chinese medicine, the stomach, where food goes, is thought of as a cauldron, and beneath the cauldron burns the fire from the kidneys and urinary bladder meridian. Under normal circumstances, the fire burns strong and is able to break down the food inside the cauldron to be utilized for nourishment throughout the body. In Winter, because the temperature outside is very cold, the ability of the kidneys to burn strong weakens; therefore, the fire is low. When cold and raw food such as salads are dumped into the cauldron, they literally put out the low fire. They require much more heat in the cauldron which the low burning fire below cannot supply. Nutrients from the cold raw veggies are not able to be processed. The result is poor digestion, but more importantly, undigested food.

What should we be eating in Winter? Glad you asked! Have you stopped to notice that people start to ingest more things with warming spices? It starts around Thanksgiving with pumpkin spices such as nutmeg, cinnamon, cloves, and ginger. These are all energetically warm spices and entirely appropriate to be eaten as the months start getting colder.

The way to think of this is that it is all about balance. If it's cold outside, you want to be eating more warm and hot foods. And *vice versa*. During Summer, foods such as watermelon and cucumbers are much more appropriate. Energetically and temperature-wise, these are cold foods. But for Winter, soups and stews are good choices. You want to eat anything that is warmed or heated gradually. It is a great time to be using a crock pot. Veggies and whatever you decide to eat should be at least stir fried or cooked all the way through. Congee, a rice dish that is slow cooked on low with lots of liquid, so that it turns the rice almost to mush, is a great dish for Winter. It is nourishing and easy on the digestion. In fact, the more simply you make the digestion process during Winter, the better it is for your body. Remember, the fire beneath the cauldron is low, and it has a more difficult time burning. By eating foods closer to already being digested, you are helping to keep that fire burning.

The taste of Winter and the corresponding kidney meridian is salty. Certain foods, such as soy sauce, miso, seaweeds, millet, and barley are salty naturally. There are also certain foods, such as ham, which are salted as a form of preservation. Adding salt to food, for flavor or preservation is o.k. but do so sparingly. The other things to focus on during Winter are warming foods. Remember, Chinese medicine is all about balance. Warm spices and foods include, but are not limited to, cloves, fenugreek seeds, fennel seeds, anise seeds, black peppercorn, ginger, cinnamon bark, walnuts, black beans, onions, garlic, chives, scallions, leeks, quinoa, chicken, lamb, trout, and salmon. Incorporating both salty and warming foods into the diet during Winter, without overdoing it, can be beneficial for your digestion. And by all means, continue making soups, stews, and slow-cooked nourishing foods.

Fear is the emotion of Winter. Fear is a natural response to a known threat. There is a good reason to be fearful when there is an apparent threat. It is the body's innate ability to put itself in fight or flight mode and keep us safe. From predators. From serious threats. There are not very many of these in our modern culture. No, in our modern culture we tend to sweat the small things. The things that seem large to us at the time. *"Where is our next meal coming from?"* is not a typical question for the majority of Americans. (Although I recognize it is for some.) The questions we ask in our day are more along the lines of, *"If I order these vitamins from California, how long will it take them to show up at my door?"* This is not exactly life threatening or serious. I mention this because we have become a culture of focusing on the minutiae. We expect things immediately and get frustrated and depressed easily and often when our expectations are not met. We have also become a culture of fearing the unknown. In fact, fear has become a way of life for entire populations of people. If nothing is apparently dangerous, some of us invent things that could be dangerous. This is pointed out to help you distinguish real threats *vs.* imagined ones. Not having enough food to eat is a real threat. Getting frustrated about not knowing what you want to eat for dinner is an imagined threat. Understand the difference and work to fix the things in your life that are not working.

What types of behaviors/activities could you be adding to your Winter routine?

* Slow down. I mean that in a quite literal sense. The Holidays which happen to occur in December in the northern hemisphere, are a hectic, busy time. That is because we make it so. Keep your Winter holidays simple and sweet. Enjoy time with a small group instead of hosting big gatherings. If you want to gather in large groups, do it at the most yang time of the year, Summer.

* Foods in the Winter are all slow cooked. Think hearty, wholesome foods. I cannot stress this point enough. It is a great time to be doing home-cooked meals.

* Start an indoor activity. I think Winter is an excellent time to begin a simple new activity. The inwardness

of the season lends itself to taking on something you have never experienced before. Have you been meaning to take a class on painting? Are you interested in learning a new musical instrument? Winter is the season.

* Enjoy the beauty of the season. In the beginning, after the first snowfall, I hear people talking about the beauty. Towards the end of the season, I mostly hear people who cannot wait for the next season. I challenge and encourage you to keep the magic of the beauty all season long.

* Whatever climate you have, enjoy the peace and stillness all season.

* Stay active but allow yourself some time for rest. Remember, Winter is a time when we need extra sleep. If we do not cultivate periods of stillness and rest, our bodies will get confused about how to achieve this at night.

* Listen to the silence. Sounds contradictory, but this time of year lends itself to a completely magnificent silence. Animals are peaceful and quiet, and in the silence, we have an opportunity to dream big.

* With longer dark hours, we have a chance to cultivate our own stillness and peace.

* Contemplate your fear. I am not saying to wallow in your fear. I am saying to ask yourself deep, soul searching questions about what is holding you back in life and work to shift your answers.

* What is one bad habit that you can begin to let go of? This most inward time of the year lends itself to redirecting areas of your life that need adjustment.

The New Moon

The New Moon brings with it the potential of new beginnings. In essence, it is the beginning of the lunar cycle, when everything has been stripped away and the darkness cleans the slate to start fresh. On a calendar, the New Moon happens in one day at one particular time. It is when the Moon is at its most yin aspect, when the moon is the least visible from our frame of reference on Earth. It doesn't mean the Moon isn't there, or that we do not feel her influence. The days leading up to the New Moon and a few days after can also impact us. The New Moon exerts the powerful force of completion and an intensity of letting go of what no longer serves us.

I love the energy of the New Moon for its freshness and the chance to clear out the old and welcome in the new. Make no mistake, the intensity of the New Moon can be just as powerful a force and just as emotionally unbalancing as the Full Moon. I think caught unaware of this intensity, people feel exhilarated and alive during the New Moon without really knowing why. The best way to flow with this intensity is to fully allow the letting go feeling to take root.

The period leading up to the New Moon, the waning phase, should be just that time. To wane, or to spread thin, to fizzle and let the dream from the Full Moon fade. This period of the cycle is perhaps even harder for us than the waxing phase because as a culture, we are more accustomed to a *get stuff done* mentality as opposed to *let stuff lie* mentality.

I see this difficulty in letting go with my acupuncture patients. We Americans have a stubborn streak, a hoarding mentality, if you will, of not being able *to give in* or *to give up*. It is like we are always in a battle *to hold on to*—ideas, ideology, possessions. I was shocked to learn that a huge growing industry in the United States is self-storage. People are not currently using possessions but are finding it important and necessary to hang on to their things. They are going as far as to pay someone else to store them. What is the fear? That you will never own things again? Or that the world is lacking *things* so that we must hold on to the ones we have?

The feeling of letting go, of allowing rather than forcing reminds me of a phenomenon in yoga. Getting into a pose, having it look a certain way is the easy part. Being—really *BE-ing*, in the pose requires an awareness of exactly what is. It is letting go, through the exhaling breath usually of a need or want for more. Just focusing on *WHAT IS*.

Without judgment, without anticipation, without expectation, without longing for different or better.

It is only in that awareness of *allowing*, that the pose will begin to evolve into something else. In other words, it is only in the *letting go of what is* that we create the space for what will be.

Once in a yoga class I was taking on Martha's Vineyard, I remember being in a standing, wide-legged, forward bend pose. The teacher's soothing voice, her attention to detail, her non-judgment of what any of her students looked like in the pose, her awareness of allowance lent itself to my sincere enjoyment in the absoluteness of the pose just as it was. Before I knew what was happening, the top of my head was touching my mat on the ground. Never before had I gotten to this level in this pose. It was an organic opening of possibilities. When I came out of the pose, I was not even sure if the experience had been real. So, at the end of class, I tried it again. Again, I had to concentrate on not focusing. With just pure enjoyment of how good this forward bend felt on my tight hamstrings, my spine, and my neck, again, my head made it to the ground.

It is this awareness of non-forcing, non-focusing that carries with it the potential for new beginnings. It is the time of the New Moon and the weeks leading up to it that can help us prepare. What is wonderful about the lunar cycle is that every month we can try again. The lunar cycle is the ultimate expression of our lives. It is endless in our lives—from the fresh new time of our birth, to the height of our life well-lived, until the decline and letting go as we age and prepare for death (and, in some cultures, are then reborn). I think it is the idea of potential that most fascinates me. One of the very first lessons I learned in yoga teacher training is this concept:

The only constant in life is change.

Think about it. Every single thing in nature evolves and grows into something different over time. Rocks eventually become sand. Flowers bloom and wither. People are born and die. If we count ourselves as part of nature, we too are constantly changing. Babies grow into toddlers, who then turn into children, who age into teenagers and become adults. The cycle is constantly pushing forward into some other version of itself. What you know and do as an adult is completely different from what you knew and did as a baby. Our unique evolving over time carries with it potential for anything and everything. A baby might change and grow up to be an opera singer, or a drug dealer. The potential for either is there.

With that said, the time of the New Moon is a time when I set an intention for the coming month. Who do I want to begin to change into? What energy am I going to focus on and grow? It can be a big or small intention. The intention can be the same month after month. Remember, after the New Moon, the roughly two weeks leading up to the Full Moon are about *building*. So, what is it that you want to build? In yourself? In the world?

The Waxing Moon

The Waxing Moon happens from the New Moon to the Full Moon. Day by day, the Moon becomes more visible. First a small sliver, then a half circle, then the full circle. The energy is growing. If you stop and pay attention, you can almost feel the bubbling up of this time of growth. It is a time to focus on and build your dreams. While the New Moon may signify a time of the seed being planted, the growing or Waxing Moon is a time when the seed has sprouted, and things are beginning to grow. The Waxing Moon is an exciting time in the aspect of being called to get stuff done. It is a particular call to action, roughly two weeks of the month, when the Moon's energy helps us work on a particular project or task. It is a particularly good time to announce the completion of a project. It is an excellent time to start a new or different project.

Even if you do not feel inspired or called to take a particular action, the Waxing Moon is an opportunity to daydream about a direction you would like to go. Even if it is a big dream, spend some special time during the Waxing Moon to really feel yourself already having attained the thing or situation you desire. You may have heard of the phrase,

That which we appreciate appreciates.

The Waxing Moon is an excellent time to start a gratitude journal. The more positive attention we give to the things we are grateful for, the more the things we are grateful for multiply. If you have never done a gratitude journal, it is quite simple. Set aside time (5 or 10 minutes is perfect) and make a list of everything in your life that brings you joy. If you are having a difficult day, and it feels like there is nothing that is making you joyful, all the better! Your list can be simple with entries like *"I am grateful for socks on my feet"* or, *"I am grateful the Sun made an appearance today."* When we start to pay attention and notice all that is going well, suddenly things that are going well happen more frequently. If you do not believe me, try it for yourself.

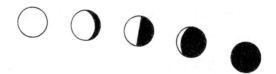

The Full Moon

Did you ever wonder where the word *lunatic* came
from? Luna is another word for moon, and people with
a strong sensitivity around the Full Moon were labeled
lunatics. These people have more difficulty sleeping
during the Full Moon, or days leading up to it. And,
they are adversely affected by the Moon's energy—short
tempered and easily emotional. The effects of the Moon
when it is in its full aspect are real and documented.
More babies are born around the Full Moon; more
suicides and homicides happen around the Full Moon.
There is a sense that everything is just a bit more
amplified—as if the volume of the Earth has been turned
up.

The Full Moon is the height of the lunar cycle. It is
when cosmic energy is at its apex. Whatever has been
building in the waxing cycle leading up to the Full Moon
is now at its completion. It is when cosmic energy is

literally bursting at the seams, and we creatives get a moment to step back and admire our hard work. The Full Moon represents the mother aspect in Celtic tradition—specifically the pregnant mother who is just about to give birth or has just given birth. The Full Moon time reminds us to show gratitude and thanks for the completion of our projects. It gives us the chance to acknowledge and respect the idea of planting a seed at the New Moon and watching it grow.

Like the New Moon, the Full Moon too can be a time of new beginnings but most likely on a bigger scale in terms of a lunar rhythm. New projects started on a Full Moon will get a full 28-day cycle to manifest. With respect to the lunar cycle, the Full Moon is an excellent time to make a list of the accomplishments and achievements since the last Full Moon. That which we appreciate appreciates, and the Full Moon reminds us to be grateful and appreciate the positives. Like our furred brothers and sisters, the wolves, the Full Moon may be a wonderful time for you to howl and rejoice in all you have done.

The Moon itself reflects its biggest and brightest light on our darkness and shortcomings. Therefore, the Full Moon is an excellent time to access and decide what layers of our shadow selves we need to next uncover.

With the guidance and light of the Full Moon, our dark human-ness does not appear scary or overwhelming. In the gentle glow of the Moon's light, we can more easily peel back the next layer of old unhealed wounds. Because it is the Sun's rays that light the Full Moon, honoring and thanking the Sun and the Moon during the Full Moon can be particularly healing and fulfilling. In yoga, Sun salutations are particularly appropriate but also check out Moon salutations. (See resources in the back of the book.)

The way I like to think of Full Moon energy is like a Thanksgiving meal. Roughly 14 days before the Full Moon, at the New Moon, you are just starting out with ingredients and recipes for the feast. These are the rough blueprints of a plan in mind. As the Moon waxes and fills, the ingredients are being added to recipes; sauces are prepared and tested; you begin to plan the table setting. A few days before the Full Moon (Thanksgiving Day) the tension and energy in the household build as the host/hostess wants everything looking, smelling, and tasting its best. On the Full Moon, the meal is offered in its completion, and the guests enjoy the fruits of all the work and preparation that began the cycle. Thanks and honor are given for every aspect of the meal, including the animals that were sacrificed. Of course, the clean-up after begins the next phase of the cycle, or waning phase. The host/hostess finally has a chance to let down their hair and revel in knowing they put their best into the process. The slate is wiped clean during the waning phase in preparation for another meal plan. At the New Moon, the cycle begins again.

The Waning Moon

During the time from Full Moon to New Moon, it is decreasing in visibility. This is called the Waning Moon. The energy during this time emphasizes letting go. It is an excellent time to step back from any projects, and while I do not recommend that you *stop* working on them, the energy at this two-week cycle is more about surrender. *Allowance* is another word I like to describe this time. You allow things to flow along, as they have been, without pushing hard for change. In yoga practice there is a difficult pose that we do at the end of every class. It is called Sivasana, or Corpse pose. If someone were to walk in on a class during Corpse pose, it would appear that everyone was napping. The pose is done lying down supine (face up) with arms and legs spread out and eyes shut. In fact, I have had students actually fall asleep during Corpse pose. When I introduce the pose to beginners, I explain that this pose is the pinnacle of all the other more active poses. It is when the body gets a chance to incorporate and assimilate the healing energy of the rest of the class. Corpse pose allows for the expansiveness that happens after the body moves through other postures. In this respect, it is one of the most important poses. Also, it can be one of the most difficult. The pose is held for a minimum of 10 minutes, and during that time, people who do not yet know how to surrender can struggle. When I am in Corpse pose and my body is completely at rest, my mind thinks it is time to take flight. I am met with a barrage of lists and thoughts that float around and will not settle. If the rest of my day is busy, Corpse pose can be challenging because my brain is telling me to get up and move.

Corpse pose reminds me of this waning time of the moon. Like all of nature, there is balance. A time for play and a time for rest. The Waning Moon is more so a time of rest. During the Waning Moon, the energy supports a clearing or washing away of the old. In fact, you may find that any difficult cleaning projects will go a lot smoother during a Waning Moon phase. Is there a closet you are wanting to clear out? Do you want to start cleaning up the garage? Do it during the Waning Moon phase. The energy of this time will support and help you. So you see, I am not suggesting that you should not be active nor start new projects during a Waning Moon. But I am saying that the Moon energy will support you best if you carefully pick and choose what projects to focus on. Did you ever have one of those days where a cleaning project just feels monumentally impossible? If you stop and look at a calendar, I would bet you are not in a waning phase.

There is one more aspect I want to offer regarding a waning cycle. Rest, relaxation, and *doing nothing,* are just as important as *doing something.* There is a large faction of our American population who have a difficult time sitting still. And, there is also a large portion of our culture who have a difficult time sleeping at night. Our bodies are not robots. There is not one switch that turns us on and turns us off. Learning how to be still and rest throughout the day will lend itself to being able to sleep more easily at night.

> **If we are not always focused on doing,
> we can be largely more focused on being.**

Being present for one another is why we are here. Helping others along, just by the simple act of being the unique you that you are, is extraordinarily valuable. Have you ever spent time with someone who has suffered a loss? Sure, you can make them meals, you can help by cleaning their house, you can run errands at the store.

But the simple act of sitting with them, in their grief, really listening to them, if they want to speak, is more healing and nurturing and loving that anything else you could *do*.

❧

As I close this book and review the information I have shared, I hope that it will bring you closer to your own awareness and reverence for the celestial rhythms and seasons in your area. We only inhabit this home we call Earth for a short time. I hope you will use some of the tools and tricks I have shared here to make your walk through this life not only more balanced, but also easier. Mother Nature, in all of her majesty, has much to teach us if we are willing to stop and listen.

Namaste,

   Michelle

Additional Resources

Andrews, Ted. *Nature-Speak: Signs, Omens and Message in Nature.* Dragonhawk Publishing, 2004.
> This book is a more serious dive into the natural rhythms of the seasons. The author is quite knowledgeable about rites and rituals around the seasons from a Native American standpoint. Like his popular book, *Animal Speak,* this book defines specific energy of the plants, trees, and the wisdom they share.

Cornell, Laura J. *Moon Salutations, Women's Journey Through Yoga to Healing, Power and Peace.* Divine Feminine Yoga, 2019.
> This book was written by my mentor, Laura Cornell. It is a fantastic exploration of the feminine side of yoga and the mysteries of the moon.

Hadady, Letha. *Asian Health Secrets: The Complete Guide to Asian Herbal Medicine.* Crown Publishers, 1996.
> This book is an easy introduction to Asian patent herbal medicine. The reason I like and use it is because it is written from the perspective of the practitioner with an intricate understanding of the balancing principle as it applies to Chinese medicine. It is like a trip to Chinatown.

Maciocia, Giovanni. *The Foundations of Chinese Medicine: A Comprehensive Text for Acupuncturists and Herbalists.* Churchill Livingstone Publishers, 1989.
> This is a required text for a degree in Chinese medicine. The author is a world-renowned authority on the principles of

Chinese medicine. I still use this text even after 20 years of practice.

Ingerman, Sandra. *Walking in Light: The Everyday Empowerment of a Shamanic Life.* Sounds True, 2014.

I have taken Sandra's online classes in Shamanism and enjoy several of her books. This is my favorite—a must for anyone interested in shamanism and the natural world.

Paungger, Johanna and Poppe, Thomas. *Moon Time: The Art of Harmony with Nature and Lunar Cycles* (1995 translated from German by David Pendlebury). Barnes and Noble Books, 1996.

This book opened up the world of Moon energy for me. It has some surprising practical recommendations, like best days to schedule a surgery.

Pitchford, Paul. *Healing with Whole Foods: Asian Traditions and Modern Nutrition.* North Atlantic Books, 2002.

This book is a serious dive into healthy eating. Everyone should own a copy and use it.

www.mygoddesspath.com. Online resource.

My dear friend and mentor, Yukiko Amaya, is a priestess and healer in the tradition of Avalon. I am currently studying with her in a year-long initiation of the seasonal goddess energies.

www.youtube.com. You Tube Channel: *Yoga with Adrienne.* Online resource.

I recommend this channel several times a week as a gentle introduction to yoga basics. She offers an extensive free library of yoga sessions which can be done in the privacy of your living room.

About the Author

Michelle's personal and professional mission as an acupuncturist and as a yoga instructor is to help you in your journey to optimal health.

In 1989, Michelle earned her bachelor's degree at Penn State. A major in women's studies fueled her passion for women's health. Her master's degree in acupuncture and Chinese herbology from Meiji College of Oriental Medicine in San Francisco, CA was completed in 1998. While on the west coast, she attended a 500-hour yoga teacher training to earn industry certification as a Registered Yoga Instructor (RYT). She has served as a practitioner of Traditional Chinese Medicine (TCM) herbology and acupuncture for over 20 years. As a yoga instructor she taught in a variety of sites in Colorado and Western Pennsylvania including Latrobe Hospital, Ligonier YMCA, several studios, gyms, private clubs, and homes.

In 2014, she and her family moved to the Western Slope of Colorado, where she worked in an integrative, alternative clinic. During that time, she extended her yoga teaching certification to include Pilates.

Following her recent return to Western Pennsylvania, her active acupuncture practice serves past patients and new patients. Michelle has successfully treated thousands of patients of all ages and medical issues.

From her studies with a practicing shaman, she has grown her love of shamanism. This book embodies her deep respect and understanding of the rocks, plants, trees, and animals of the natural world that we share on this planet. This, in addition to Chinese medicine, acupuncture, and yoga, are tools that combine with her empathy, to uniquely guide you on your path toward balance with the natural world and a deeper connection with spirit on your path to wellness.

Along with their father, George Clark, she birthed and raised two happy healthy teenage boys, Aidan and Evan.

CPSIA information can be obtained
at www.ICGtesting.com
Printed in the USA
BVHW062110310821
615694BV00015B/1155

9 780941 461023